The Seniors' Workout

Stretches, Exercises & Aerobics

Dr. Larry McConnell

First Edition 2015
ISBN-13: 978-1505639698

Photographs by Katherine Caine

Note: The websites listed in the text were verified on January 04, 2015.

For the couch potatoes
seeking a better way

Behind The Scenes

My thanks to Katherine Caine, the photographer who did the photo shoot and edited all the images. Katherine managed this demanding project with enthusiasm, patience and good humour. The results are a tribute to her exceptional professionalism.

My love, admiration and thanks to Sharon Mulroney. Like all my books, this one would never have come to fruition without my wife's assistance. I am particularly thankful for her technical support and endless patience with the editing process.

Lastly, three cheers for our dog, Stella. I appreciate her modelling efforts even though she was unable to camouflage her boredom. Stella is a happy hound who enjoys good food, exercise, people and sleep. I say that makes her a pretty good role model.

Contents

INTRODUCTION

A FEW WORDS ABOUT EXERCISE   1

THE HUNCHBACK   4

THE TUMMY TONER   6

THE BELLY CRUNCHER   7

THE ROLLY POLLY   8

THE CIRCLE DANCE & HAMSTER   9

THE BIG STRETCH   11

THE LEG TWISTERS   12

THE BICYCLE   16

THE TOE GRABBER   18

THE WRIST FLEXOR   19

OVER THE TOP   21

THE BALANCE BEAM & LONG JOHN SILVER   23

THE WALL LEANER   28

THE TOE BUSTER   30

LOOSE AS A GOOSE   32

THE NECK BENDER   34

BELLY DANCING   36

THE PUNTER   37

PUMPING IRON   38

THE HEEL PULLER   42

THE SHRUG   44

THE YOGA MAN   45

THE BACK CRUNCHER & SUPERMAN   46

THE TURTLE   47

THE KNEE BENDER   48

HUFFING AND PUFFING   51

INTRODUCTION

I turned seventy years old last year in great shape. I have been a fitness buff my whole life. My father was a gifted athlete who excelled in hockey, rowing and boxing. He was teaching me how to work out before I even started school. In those days, the body builder, Charles Atlas, was the man, but we did not own any weights so I was taught to do calisthenics and run my butt off to keep in shape. I loved to run. In grade school I would run laps around a vacant lot across from the school for at least an hour at lunchtime and still manage to be the teacher's biggest challenge for the rest of the afternoon. In today's world that sort of behaviour gets one labeled ADHD.

I also was active in any sport I got the opportunity to play. Such was my experience throughout my school years. As I grew older my exercise routines and choice of sports changed, but I always kept in shape. I let up for a year or two in graduate school, but after graduation got right back at it. This lifelong devotion to physical training has left me with the strength, mobility, flexibility and endurance to continue pursuing an extremely active lifestyle as I age.

I want to share my fitness program with you but first, a word of caution. Obviously I have no way of knowing the physical condition of any reader. What I do know is we are all different when it comes to exercise. A routine that works for one person may prove a disaster for the next one. So consult with your health care professional before you try any of the training methods outlined here. If you have been inactive and plan to start a physical conditioning program, ask your medical doctor about getting a stress test and/or an EKG or even an echocardiogram. Furthermore, even if you get the green light to go ahead, proceed at a slow pace. My fitness program, including the aerobic component, runs over two hours. It takes time to build up that amount of endurance.

Finally, remember that the notion 'no pain no gain' is a foolish one, especially in relation to people our ages. We have to cope with enough aches and pains without adding a few more by overextending ourselves. So take it easy. A nice, even pace where you enjoy your workout should be the goal. You are trying to remain fit, not qualify for the Olympics.

A Few Words About Exercise

I have read countless scientific studies concerned with testing the effect of exercise on people of all shapes and sizes. These studies report consistent results. Exercise is good for you irrespective of age, gender, weight or athletic ability. It even can help people with health issues. For example, exercise has been shown to reduce arterial stiffness. This is a relevant finding for older folks because arterial stiffness tends to occur with age and increases the risk of cardiovascular problems.[1] Yet the benefits are not limited to physical health. Exercise also can enrich psychological well-being and augment one's mental capacities. In fact, there is even evidence suggesting exercise may reduce the risk of dementia and slow its progression.[2] Indeed exercise, along with genes, good nutrition and limited stress, is a principal contributor to a long and healthy life. In contrast, a sedentary lifestyle leaves one with a weakened body where physical endurance wanes, strength fades, flexibility diminishes, and mobility becomes more and more limited.

Exercise is fun and has a good payoff, but it does have some limitations. For instance, it is not very useful as a weight loss tool. You are better off following the 'eat less' maxim when trying to lose weight. Think about it. You have to drop 3,500 calories to lose a pound. That means for each pound you wish to lose, you must eat 3,500 calories less or work off 3,500 calories. So if you want to drop a pound in a week, you either reduce your daily food intake by 500 calories or work out five times a week burning 700 calories each session. If you choose the latter route, be prepared to spend a lot of time working out. For example, if you weigh

[1] See http://www.ncbi.nlm.nih.gov/pmc/articles/PMC2713633/ This was a particularly impressive outcome as the sample group was older adults with type 2 diabetes complicated by comorbid hypertension and hyperlipidemia. Also see *Diabetes Care*, 2009 August; 32(8): 1531–1535.

[2] See http://newsnetwork.mayoclinic.org/discussion/tuesday-q-a-regular-physical-exercise-has-powerful-effect-on-brain-health. You may want to browse the *Mayo Clinic* website as it reports on numerous studies related to the advantages of exercise.

about 160 pounds and your exercise of choice is swimming, you will have to swim laps for an hour and forty minutes, five times a week to burn off the 3,500 calories. That means more than eight hours a week in the pool. I am sure it can be done, but it may turn you into a prune.[3] No question about it, the wiser and easier choice is to consume less food.

It also is not a good idea to view exercise as a justification for eating more snacks. Some people with a tendency to overeat set up food as a reward for completing an exercise session. Their reasoning runs something like this: 'Well my workout was top-notch, so now I can enjoy a treat without worrying about the extra calories'. Be careful. Regular exercise does leave you a little slack when it comes to eating more, but not much. Chances are you have no idea how many calories you burned with the exercise, and you are probably overestimating the amount you can eat that is equivalent to the calories you just burned off. Pity the poor people who finish their forty-minute, low-impact aerobics class and reward themselves with a small bag of chips and a pop. The good news is their aerobic session burned off around two hundred and fifty calories.[4] The bad news is their 'little reward' amounted to more than three hundred calories. Oops! Back to the gym.

So if you want to reward yourself for sticking to an exercise regime, make it a non-food reward. The fact is, exercise is not about losing weight or making room for more food. Sure it can be one of many factors helping you to maintain good body weight, but its real benefits lie elsewhere. Exercise is the vehicle for building and maintaining body strength, flexibility, mobility and endurance. It also increases your energy levels and helps you to look and to feel good. These sound like pretty good incentives to me.

---

[3] I am an avid swimmer in the winter but never come close to spending that kind of time in the pool.
[4] See http://www.mayoclinic.com/health/exercise/SM00109 for the number of calories burned per hour doing various activities.

Most mornings I get out of bed between eight and eight-thirty. I wash up, feed the dog and let her out, bring my wife breakfast (in bed no less), pour myself a glass of orange juice and head downstairs to my cave in the basement. If you are going to work out indoors, it is wise to find a place in your house or apartment where you can spend time without interruptions. My workout regime requires little space and no equipment apart from two small eight-pound barbells. I also have a small mat down on the rug to make it more comfortable for my old body. The workout portion of my fitness program involves a significant amount of stretching, low tempo exercises and some strength training. It lasts a little longer than an hour. I work through the entire training session in my bare feet without employing any special breathing techniques. The radio is always on while I am working out. I usually listen to country music or a current affairs program on the CBC.[5] This helps to keep my mind occupied while I engage in mindless activity.

In the detailed descriptions that follow, I describe the exercises and stretches in the order I perform them in my routine. However, there is nothing special about this sequence so customize the routine to your preferences. The accompanying pictures will help you gain a better idea of the body position for each exercise and stretch. The reproductions are authentic, but I am neither a professional trainer nor a model, so the form is rather minimalist, although good enough to get the job done. Remember, we are old folks. It is not about 'the look'. It is all about getting down on the floor and getting 'er done. So let's get at it.

---

[5] The CBC is Canada's publically funded radio and television station.

The Hunchback

This first stretch is for your back and spine. I am a very keen golfer, so a durable back is of eminent importance to me. I have learned to do numerous types of stretches for my wonky back, but in my judgment none of them does the trick quite like this one.[6] I perform it faithfully before every round of golf I play. This stretch is felt primarily in the lower back. Here is how it works:

- Get down on the mat on your hands and knees.
- Keep your thighs about six inches (15 cm) apart and perpendicular to the mat.
- Your hands should be palms down on the mat about twelve inches (30 cm) in front of your knees.
- Keep your elbows straight and your eyes focussed on the mat.
- Now move your chin toward your chest and hunch your back (Fig.1).

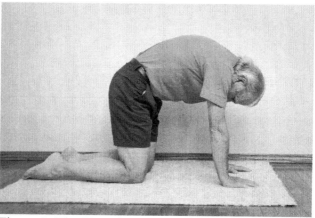

Figure 1. The Hunchback (a)

---

[6] Some of the stretches I describe here can be found on the *Canadian Centre for Occupational Health and Safety* website.
See http://www.ccohs.ca/oshanswers/psychosocial/backexercises.html

4

- Hold this position for about ten seconds.
- Slowly return your head and back to the original position and pause for a second.
- Then move your head up slightly, drop your belly down and curve your lower back so it forms an arc (Fig.2).

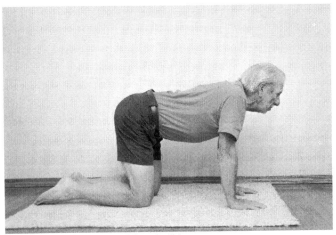

Figure 2. The Hunchback (b)

- Hold this position for about ten seconds.
- Do eight to ten repetitions of the overall sequence.

The Tummy Toner

Some keeners may be tempted to skip this exercise deeming it too tame to be beneficial. However, I encourage you to do it as a gentle warm-up for more vigorous stretches and exercises designed to strengthen your back and tighten up your stomach muscles. It does not require much effort and takes only a few minutes. It also is a particularly good starter for older folks who are just beginning to exercise their back and stomach muscles.

- Lie down on your back.
- Place your hands palms down on the mat under the lower part of your back.
- Keep the left leg relaxed and outstretched on the mat.
- Slowly raise the right leg until it is parallel to the mat from the knee to the heel (Fig. 3).

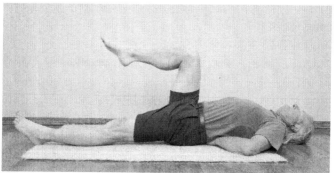

Figure 3. The Tummy Toner

- Hold this position for five or six seconds.
- Repeat the procedure with your left leg.
- Repeat the stretch five or six times with each leg.

The Belly Cruncher

I am not a big fan of traditional sit-ups. They place too much strain on the back even when done with the knees bent or both feet up on a chair. The Belly Cruncher is a modified alternative to the conventional sit-up. It is one of two exercises I do aimed directly at my stomach muscles. They seem to work as my stomach is quite firm. The big plus? There is less risk to my temperamental back.

- Keep your hands on the mat palms down under your spine just above your hips.
- Raise your shoulders and drop your chin toward your chest (Fig. 4).

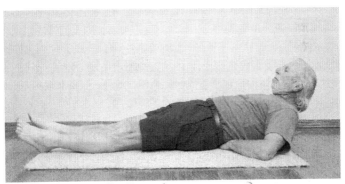

Figure 4. The Belly Cruncher

- Hold this position for five or six seconds. Do not force it.
- While holding the position, try turning your neck back and forth from left to right.
- Slowly lower your head and shoulders back to the floor.
- Repeat twenty-five times.

The Rolly Polly

This is another stretch for my back. It is an oldie but a goodie. I started doing it in high school. It is low impact but it does help to extend my back muscles. I have added a turning motion to the upright position that helps to loosen my neck muscles.

- Remain on your back outstretched on the mat.
- Pull up both your knees and wrap your arms around them.
- Now pull your knees up as far as possible toward your chest (Fig.5).

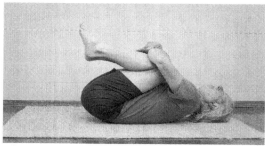

Figure 5. The Rolly Polly (a)

- Hold this position for ten seconds.
- Now bring your head and shoulders up toward your knees (Fig.6).

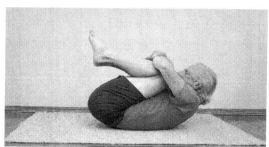

Figure 6. The Rolly Polly (b)

- Hold this position for about ten seconds.
- You also can work your neck in this position by slowly turning it from left to right.
- Return your head to the mat and repeat this sequence four or five times.

The Circle Dance & Hamster.

These are two more movements to practice while you are lying down on your back. The Circle Dance helps to increase extension and flexibility around the buttocks and groin areas. The Hamster is directed at the hamstrings which are a group of tendons located at the back of the thighs. They are hard at work flexing our knees and extending our hips when we are running, jumping, walking or climbing stairs. It is not uncommon to lose some flexibility here as we age, but these two stretches can help slow down the process. Working to maintain muscle extension capacity is also a good way to protect your hamstrings and groin areas from injuries. If this is your first attempt at these moves, I suggest you proceed at a gradual pace to avoid pulling any muscle.

- Take up the position as shown in Figure 5.
- Let go of your left knee and rest your left leg straight out along the floor.
- Keep holding the right knee with both hands.
- Slowly rotate the knee clockwise in an increasingly wider circle (Fig.7)

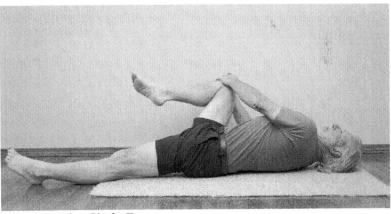

Figure 7. The Circle Dance

- After several rotations, change direction and do several more rotations counter-clockwise.

9

- Now move your hands down to where you can lock your fingers behind your right thigh.
  Gently pull your right leg up until it is at least perpendicular to your body (Fig.8).

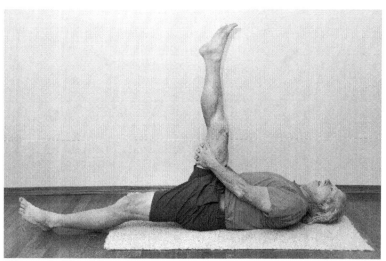

Figure 8. The Hamster

- Try to keep the right leg reasonably straight at the knee.
- Hold this position for ten seconds.
- Now go through the *Circle Dance* and *Hamster* with the left leg.

Try to repeat the complete routine two or three times with each leg. You can enhance the Hamster by pointing your toes at your face. This is a good way to stretch your calves. You can also rotate your foot while it is in the air to give your ankle a workout.

The Big Stretch

Take a breather with the Big Stretch. There is no real purpose to this stretch other than to keep you loose and give you a good feeling. Simply lie on your back and stretch out your arms and legs as far as they will go (Fig. 9). Hold the position for ten or fifteen seconds.

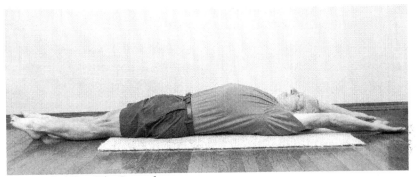

Figure 9. The Big Stretch

When you have completed the Big Stretch, go back to the Belly Cruncher exercise (Fig. 4). Follow the original routine except this time, raise your elbows up off the floor. In other words, you raise your head, shoulders and *elbows* while moving your chin toward your collarbone. Do twenty-five more belly crunchers in this way.

The Leg Twisters

Seniors want to retain their capacity to get around with ease. Mobility is a big deal. Indeed as we age, our quality of life is significantly influenced by our level of mobility which, in turn, is largely determined by the condition of our legs and feet. In this regard, I am a firm believer in the 'use it or lose it' principle. If you are a notorious couch potato, you significantly increase the odds your mobility and flexibility will reduce a lot more rapidly as you age. In contrast, with regular exercise there is no reason for you to experience a dramatic reduction in your capacity to move around. With this in mind, I use the leg twisters in my routine to help maintain strength and flexibility in my legs. I have a separate routine for my ankles and feet which I describe later in this section. There are two sets of leg twisters. Here is the first one.

- Lie on the mat on your back with your legs outstretched along the floor.
- Place your right arm along the floor, even with your shoulder.
- Grab your right knee on the outside with your left hand.
- Pull the knee toward your left hip until the toes on your right foot are touching the mat by the outside of your left knee (Fig. 10).

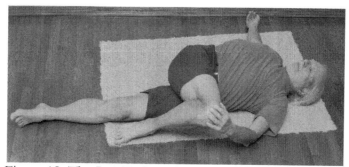

Figure 10. The Leg Twister (1a)

- Push down on your knee until your left elbow is on the floor.
- Hold this position for five to eight seconds.

- Repeat the same stretch using your right arm and left knee.
- Do the complete set three times.

Now return to the original position.
- Join your feet at the soles and then pull them toward your crotch.
- Raise your shoulders and head up toward your feet (Fig. 11).

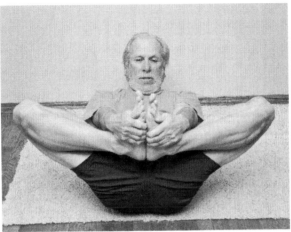

Figure 11. The Leg Twister (1b)

- Push down on your feet while keeping your knees as far apart as possible.
- Hold this position for ten seconds.
- Repeat three times.

Now return to the original position on your back to start the second set of leg twisters.
- Lift your left leg and grab the sole of your left foot with your right hand.
- Rest your left hand and forearm along the outside of your left calf and thigh for support.
- Pull your left foot and ankle toward your head until you feel a pull in your buttock.

- Raise your head from the floor until your nose is touching your left knee (Fig.12).

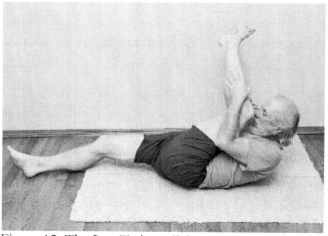

Figure 12. The Leg Twister (2a)

- Hold this position for about ten seconds.
- Now raise your right leg up beside the left one.
- Rest the back of your right lower calf on top of your left knee.
- Wrap both hands around the left leg just below the knee (Fig. 13).

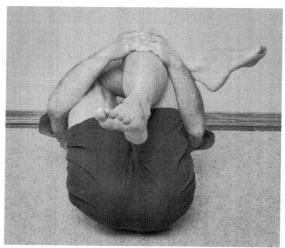

Figure 13. The Leg Twister (2b)

- Pull your left knee in the direction of your face.
- You will feel the stretch in your lower back and right buttock.
- Now raise your head and shoulders toward your right knee (Fig. 14).

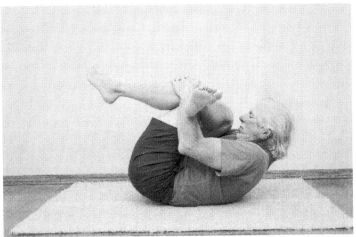

Figure 14. The Leg Twister (2c)

- Hold this position for ten seconds.
- Repeat the exercise, this time lifting your right leg and grabbing the sole of your right foot with your left hand.
- Repeat the series two or three times with each leg.

The Bicycle

We are going to increase the tempo somewhat here. The bicycle is probably the most strenuous exercise in the overall repertoire, so adjust the pace to your level of fitness. That means a slow, steady pace if you are a beginner. The bicycle is geared to strengthening your stomach muscles, although it also can have an aerobic impact if you do it long enough at a quick pace. You want to gradually build up endurance, but there is no rush, so stop when you feel the strain or tire out. Here is how it works.

- Return to the original position lying on your back on the mat.
- Lock your fingers behind your head.
- Raise your legs and start to pump them as though you are peddling a bicycle (Fig. 15).

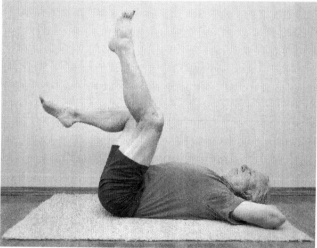

Figure 15. The Bicycle (a)

- Take a practice run by attempting to raise your head a few inches off the mat while still pedalling.
- Pedal at different speeds until you find a comfortable rhythm.
- Return your head to the mat.

- Now lift your head and twist it as close as you can to your left knee while you peddle. (Fig.16).

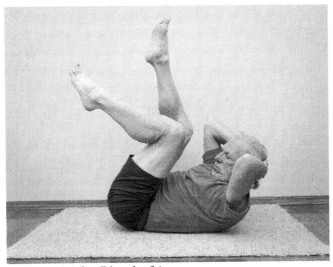

Figure 16. The Bicycle (b)

- Put your head back on the mat; then come up again twisting your head as far as you can toward the right knee.
- Return your head to the mat.
- Continue this drill alternately reaching for the left and right knees.
- The long range goal is one hundred repetitions.

This is a difficult exercise for the beginner, so obviously it would be foolish to try and complete one hundred repetitions at the start. You may want to begin with ten or twenty. However, if you stick with it, you will discover it does not take long to get to the point where you can do over a hundred repetitions without feeling significant discomfort. As you get better at this exercise you can work at increasing the tempo, pulling your head up closer and closer to your knees, and doing more repetitions. It is a good one for tightening up the ol' gut.

The Toe Grabber

This stretch is good for the back, knees, toes and hamstrings. It does tug at the knees when done properly.

- Stretch your right leg straight out along the mat.
- Bring the sole of your left foot up against the inside of the right knee and thigh.
- Make sure the right leg remains straight out at the knee.
- Bending from the waist, reach for the toes on your right foot with both hands.
- Pull the toes back toward your waist (Fig. 17).

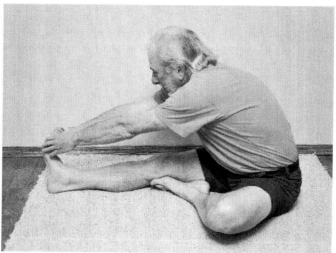

Figure 17. The Toe Grabber

- Hold this position for thirty seconds.
- Repeat the process with your left leg extended straight out along the mat.
- Repeat once more with each leg.

The Wrist Flexor

This stretch is designed to increase flexibility in your wrist and fingers. The stretch is easy to do, but it does put a fair amount of pressure on the joints of your fingers. If you have arthritis in your hands, proceed with caution until you determine whether or not it is painless and helpful.

- Stand on the mat with your feet a few centimetres/inches apart.
- Move the left foot forward about six inches (15 cm).
- Bend your right knee until you feel pressure just above the heel.
- Raise your right arm bending it at the elbow.
- The palm of your right hand should be facing down.
- Turn your wrist so that the fingers are pointing straight ahead.
- Place your left hand over the knuckles of your right hand and press down (Fig. 18).

Stella says, 'If only I had fingers.'

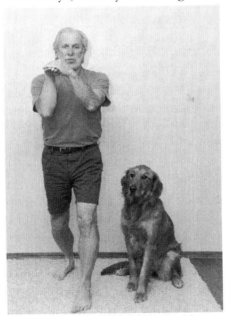

Figure 18. The Wrist Flexor (a)

- Maintain this position for about six seconds.
- Remaining in the same position, turn your hand over so that the palm is facing up.
- Twist your wrist until the fingers are pointing at you.
- Place your left hand across your thumb and fingers and push down (Fig. 19).

Stella says, 'But my front paws are right.'

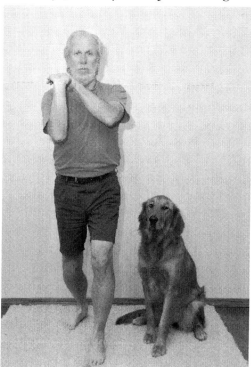

Figure 19. The Wrist Flexor (b)

- Maintain this position for about six seconds.
- Now reverse your leg position, switch arms and repeat the process with the left hand.
- Repeat the sequence twice with each hand.

Over The Top

This next stretch is one I was taught years ago by a chiropractor when I was experiencing rather painful sciatica symptoms. She described it as a simple stretch that does wonders on the preventative front. She has me convinced because I did incorporate it into my repertoire and have never experienced the pain again. Try it

- Stand on the mat with your feet about forty-five centimetres (18 ins.) apart and your hands by your sides
- Raise your right arm above your head keeping the elbow straight.
- Bending at the waist, slide your left hand down your left leg (Fig. 20).

Stella says, 'Hey, I can pose too.'

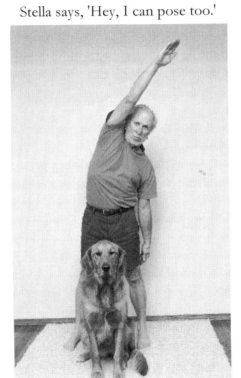

Figure 20. Over The Top

- Lean to the left as far as you can, and then hold the position for eight to ten seconds.
- Keeping the same position, move your right hand forward about thirty degrees.
- Hold this position another eight to ten seconds.
- Repeat the process with your left hand above your head and slide your right hand down your right leg.

The Wrist Flexor and Over The Top stretches work well in tandem. I usually do the Wrist Flexor with each hand twice and then switch to the Over The Top stretch doing it once to each side of my body. I repeat this combination two or three times.

The Balance Beam / Long John Silver

The next two exercises focus on balance.[7] A sense of balance is important because, among other things, it helps us to walk without staggering, climb stairs without tripping, and avoid serious falls. Unfortunately the sense of balance is somewhat compromised by the gradual loss of vision, hearing and muscle strength which most people experience in their later years. However, we can compensate for this loss by doing exercises such as the Balance Beam and Long John Silver.

I recommend a simple test to evaluate your present level of balance before you try these exercises. It is a common test you may have been asked to do when getting a medical checkup. Simply stand barefoot on the floor and then raise one of your legs about a foot in front of you. See how long you can hold that position. Do it twice with each foot and get the average to use as your baseline. I suggest you strive for a minimum of ten seconds. A tougher test is to stand with your eyes closed, and if you are right-handed, raise the right foot (the left foot if you are left-handed) about six inches off the floor putting the knee at a 45 degree angle. You are one well-balanced old timer if you can hold that position for six or seven seconds. Remember, even if you are bit shaky, over time it is possible to improve your balance by doing a few exercises.

The first one requires you to take a standard position used when practicing on a high beam. However, you remain solidly planted on the floor. You will note, Stella has passed on this one, but you should give it a go.

- Stand on the mat with your arms by your sides.
- Raise your arms straight out sideways shoulder high.

---

[7] Scott McCredie, *Balance: In Search of the Lost Sense*, Little Brown and Company, 2007. This is a good book if you are looking for more details on the importance of our sense of balance.

- Lift the left foot until your thigh is parallel to the mat (Fig. 21).

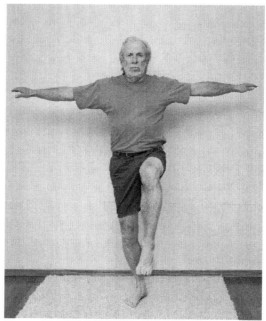

Figure 21. The Balance Beam

- Hold this position for ten or fifteen seconds before returning your foot to the mat.
- Now raise your right foot until your thigh is parallel to the mat.
- Hold this position for ten or fifteen seconds.
- Repeat the exercise three times with each foot.

The next exercise is named after the peg-legged pirate so well known by our generation. The name seems fitting since it demands the kind of balance this scoundrel no doubt required to move around his ship with only one good leg. The exercise has the added advantage of giving your knee a good stretch while you work on your balance. You may be a bit shaky when first trying this balancing act, so stand by your bed to ensure a soft landing should you topple over. Start by practicing to stand on one foot for a short period of time. Then while on one foot, attempt to raise an arm above your head. Lastly, try to take one foot in your hand and raise it behind your knee.

When you feel ready, have a go at the Long John Silver balancing act.

- Stand on the mat with your arms by your sides and bend your right knee.
- Using your right hand, take hold of the top of the right foot just above the big toe.
- Slowly raise your right foot toward your right buttock.
- Keep moving the foot back until your heel is close to your right buttock.
- Raise your left arm over your head keeping the elbow, wrist and fingers straight (Fig. 22).

Stella says, 'Booorrring.'

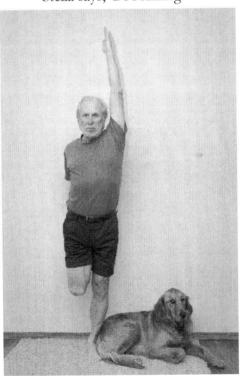

Figure 22. Long John Silver (a)

- Maintain this position for twenty seconds.

25

- Repeat the process standing on your right foot (Fig. 23).
Stella says 'Reeeeally Booorrring.'

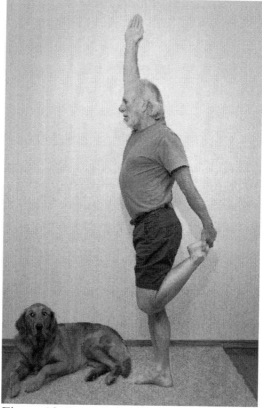

Figure 23. Long John Silver (b)

- Do the exercise two or three times on each foot.

I prefer these two exercises when it comes to working on balance, but there are other options. For example, one of my buddies likes to do what he calls the Tightrope Walk. He extends his arms straight out at his sides and pretends he is walking along a tightrope by placing one foot immediately in front of the other. He walks straight ahead for five or six metres and then returns to his starting point by walking backwards. It works. Another thing you can do is practice standing on one foot. I do this frequently when I am waiting my turn in the fairway out on the golf course. Whatever your preference, just make sure to include a few exercises in your daily routine specifically directed at balance maintenance. Once you have been doing your balance exercises for a month or two, try taking the balance test again to re-evaluate your level of balance. Obviously the goal is to get to the point where you can exceed your original baseline.

This completes the first half of the workout. This phase should take about a half hour once you become familiar with all the routines. At this point, I usually take a ten minute break to play with the dog, practice my putting or strum out a few tunes on my guitar. Then it is back to the workout. You will be standing up for the next phase.

The Wall Leaner

The next couple of exercises are for your feet. It is important to spend time stretching and exercising your feet since they play such a crucial role when it comes to maintaining mobility, which is the mainstay of your independence. If your feet are not in good shape, you will experience restrictions that are bound to have a negative impact on your overall quality of life. Plantar fasciitis, bunions, tendonitis, toenail fungus, stress fractures and warts are some of the more common foot problems that hinder mobility. Obviously, if you are experiencing any of these conditions, you should be consulting with your health professional. He or she can best advise you on how to care for your feet. If your feet are in reasonably good shape, you still should be working them with stretches and exercises for prevention purposes.[8] Here is a good stretch to start you on the road to better foot care.

The *Wall Leaner* serves a dual purpose. It gives the feet a good stretch, and it also works as a strengthening exercise. You may think the stretch is not doing much for your feet because you feel most of the pull in your calf muscles, but actually this is helpful because foot pain often originates with tight calf muscles. The strengthening part of the exercise comes from the body weight put on your arms when you lean against the wall.

- Stand a little more than a metre/yard from the wall.
- Face the wall with your feet about nine inches (23 cm) apart.
- Lift your arms about shoulder height in front of you.
- Lean forward until the palms of your hands are resting on the wall.
- Position your body so your neck, elbows, waist, and knees are straight.

---

[8] Again I stress the importance of consulting with a health professional before you start any exercise or stretching program irrespective of your physical condition or overall health.

- Now bend your elbows. Keep your waist and knees straight.
- Heels flat on the floor (Fig. 24).

Stella says, 'This is scary………….. if he falls, I'm minced meat.'

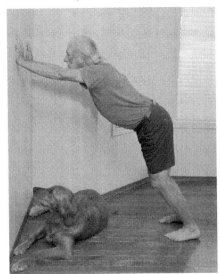

Figure 24. The Wall Leaner (a)   Figure 25. The Wall Leaner (b)

- Hold this position for ten seconds.
- Return to the original position.
- Now bend your knees while keeping your heels on the floor.
- The elbows remain straight.
- Hold this position for ten seconds (Fig. 25).
- Do ten repetitions for each position.

The Toe Buster

The Toe Buster helps to put a bit of flexibility into the joints around your toes. Most people never think to stretch or exercise their toes, but it is a good idea to keep them nimble because of the instrumental role they play in your walking stride. Painful or stiff toes definitely will slow you down. This is another multi-purpose stretch where you can stretch your Achilles tendons, which is good for your feet, while you rotate your wrists and work your toes. When the Toe Buster is done correctly, you feel pressure on the bottom of the toes and the back of the heel.

- Stand about two feet (60 cm) from the wall.
- Bring your right foot forward and press your toes up against the base of the wall.
- Rest the top of your head against the wall.
- Keeping the left leg fairly stiff, bend the right knee until it is touching the wall.
- Clench your fists (Fig. 26).

'Stella ran for cover.'

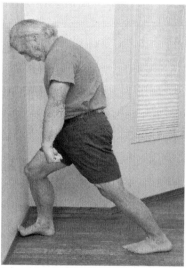

Figure 26. The Toe Buster (a)

30

- Rotate your hands to give your wrists a workout at the same time.
- Hold the position for about twenty seconds.
- Switch feet and repeat the same routine (Fig.27)

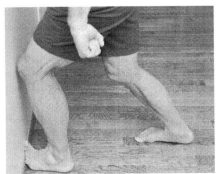

Figure 27. The Toe Buster (b)

- Repeat twice with each foot.

Loose as a Goose

This next segment in the routine concentrates on movements that help to enhance suppleness around the neck, shoulders and hips. The first is rather straightforward in that you are just swinging your arms around. It also works well as a warm-up before a swim. Try it.

- Stand on the mat with your feet about 40 cm (15 ins) apart.
- Raise your arms about shoulder height in front of you.
- Cross the arms with your left arm on top (Fig. 28).
- Start to turn the left arm counter-clockwise and the right arm clockwise.
- Rotate the arms in front of you making a complete circle (Fig. 29).

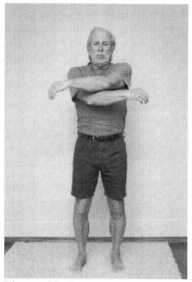 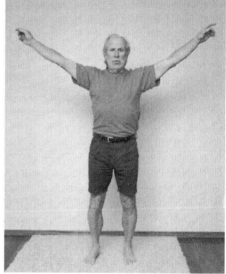

Figure 28. Loose as a Goose(a)   Figure 29. Loose as a Goose (b)

- Pick up the pace continuing for about fifteen seconds.
- Switch and turn the right arm counter-clockwise and the left arm clockwise.
- Keep the pace going for another fifteen seconds.

32

- Now keeping your feet in the same position on the mat, bring your arms down by your sides.
- Start swinging your arms backwards (Fig. 30)

'The beauty queen is back'

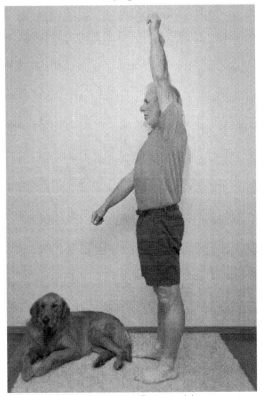

Figure30. Loose as a Goose (c)

- Quicken the pace and continue for about fifteen seconds.
- Come to a stop with the arms at your sides.
- Now start rotating them forwards.
- Quicken the pace and continue for another fifteen seconds.
- Repeat the whole set two or three times.

The Neck Bender

This is a very effective stretch for keeping the neck supple. It is a great stretch to do when you sit at a computer for extended periods of time. If you are prone to getting a stiff neck, you may find it helpful to do this stretch three or four times a day as a preventive measure. It can be done standing up or sitting down.

- Stand on the mat with your feet about 40 cm (15 ins) apart.
- Place your hands at the back of your head just above the neck.
- Lock your fingers
- Make sure your legs, back and shoulders are straight (Fig. 31)

'Stella has gone out for a jog'

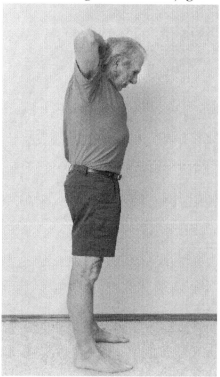

Figure 31. The Neck Bender

- Gently push your head down toward your chest. Only your head should move.
- Remain still with your chin touching the top of your chest (Fig.32).

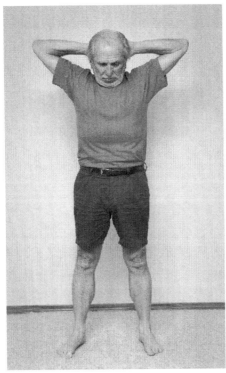

Figure 32. The Neck Bender

- Hold the position for about ten seconds.
- Slowly move your head back up to the erect position.
- Repeat the routine five times.

Belly Dancing

Now try a little *Belly Dancing*. This motion is good for developing some flexibility in the waist area. At first your movement may be somewhat restricted, but do not let that discourage you. With a little practice you will be a match for any belly dancer. Yeah right!

- Stand on the mat with your feet about 40 cm (15 ins.) apart.
- Place your hands on your hips. Keep your feet flat on the mat.
- Push your left hip forward and out (Fig.33).

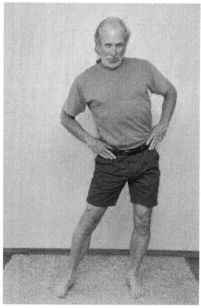

Figure 33. Belly Dancing

- Slowly begin to rotate your waist and hips clockwise while keeping your feet still.
- Move around in as wide a circle as possible.
- Keep this circular motion going for about ten seconds.
- Do the same motion in the opposite direction for ten seconds.
- Repeat the sequence two or three times.

The Punter

This is an exercise that strengthens back muscles, improves flexibility in the upper legs and helps develop better balance. I caution you to proceed slowly when learning to swing your legs in this way. Some keeners get overly enthusiastic, aim for the ceiling and end up injuring their backs. Go slowly and respect your limitations.

- Hold onto a chair with your right hand.
- Keep your left foot flat on the floor.
- Start to swing your right leg back and forth.
- Gradually increase the length of the swing.
- Swing forward high enough for the leg to be at least parallel to the floor (Fig. 34).
- Swing back until your leg is at least parallel to the floor (Fig. 35).

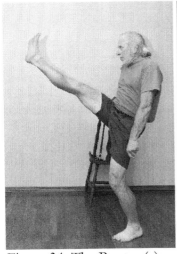 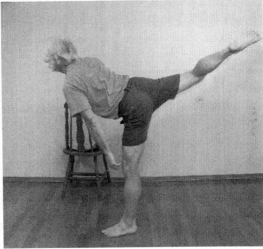

Figure 34. The Punter (a)   Figure 35. The Punter (b)

- Swing back and forth for several seconds.
- Turn the other way and hold the chair with your left hand.
- Swing your left leg back and forth in the same way.

Pumping Iron

One look at me and you can see I am no weightlifter. It is an activity that has never interested me. Even when I was a young guy, I never got into pumping iron in any serious way. That is probably one reason for my tiny arms. Nevertheless, for strengthening purposes, I do believe it is helpful to spend some time exercising with light weights. I use a pair of eight-pound barbells for ten to fifteen minutes in my workout. The routine is very simple. It will not build muscles, but it will help improve strength.

• Stand with your feet apart about 30 cm (12 ins) and your knees slightly bent.

• Hold a barbell (5 - 10 lb/2.3 - 4.5 kg) in each hand.

• The palms of your hands should be wrapped around the weights facing upward (Fig.36).

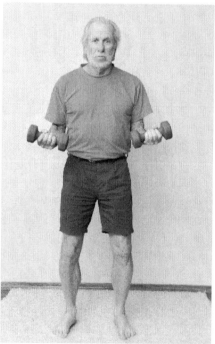

Figure 36. Bicep Curls

- Curl your arms up until the weights reach your shoulders.
- Bring the weights back down to your sides.
- Repeat this bicep curl 25 times.
- Next turn your wrist so the palms of your hands are facing down and bent toward you.
- Raise the weights in front of you shoulder high, elbows nearly straight (Fig. 37).

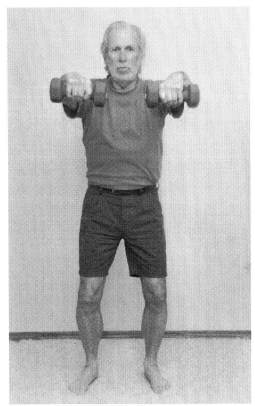

Figure 37. Stiff Arms

- Bring the weights back down to your sides.
- Repeat 5 times.
- Now turn your wrists so the palms of your hands are facing up.

- Raise the weights in front of you shoulder high, elbows nearly straight.
- Bring the weights back down to your sides.
- Repeat 5 times.
- Now turn your wrists so the palms of your hands are facing toward your sides.
- Lift the weights up from your sides until they are shoulder high.
- Keep the elbows nearly straight (Fig. 38).

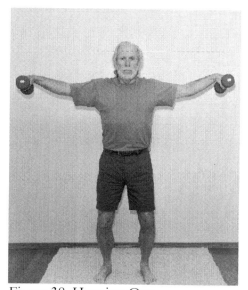 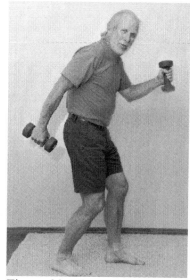

Figure 38. Hanging Out   Figure 39. The Side Swing

- Bring the weights back down to your sides.
- Repeat 5 times.
- Do the stiff arms sequence again (Fig. 37).
- Do 25 curls again (Fig. 36).
- Next hold the weights with the palms of your hands facing your sides.
- Swing your arms so that when one is up the other is down (Fig. 39).
- Repeat 26 times.

- Do 25 bicep curls again (Fig.36).
- Next hold the weights in front of your chest (Fig. 40).
- Extend your arms straight out, shoulder high (Fig. 41).

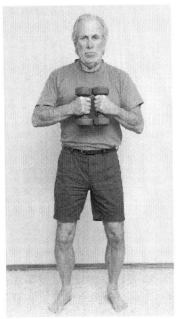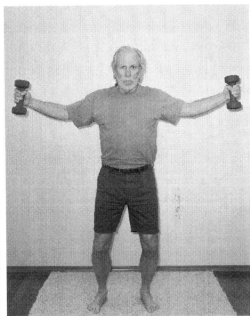

Figure 40. The Stretch (a)   Figure 41. The Stretch (b)

- Return the weights to your chest.
- Repeat 25 times.
- Do 25 bicep curls again (Fig.36).
- Do 26 side swings again (Fig. 39).

That is enough iron pumping for me. The routine has not given me bulging biceps, but it has helped me to maintain a reasonable amount of strength in my arms.

Okay. Now let us do a little more foot work.
Move to an open doorway for this next sequence of stretches.

41

The Heel Puller

I added the Heel Puller to my routine five or six years ago. It was recommended by a physiotherapist who helped me to get rid of the pain I was experiencing from heel spurs. Other people also have found the stretch helpful when they were bothered by plantar fasciitis, heel pain or Achilles tendonitis. You will certainly feel a pull in the Achilles tendon. It is best to perform this stretch in a doorway, although it can be done against a wall.

- Stand about 75 cm (30 ins) in front of an open doorway.
- Place your hands on either side of the door frame just below shoulder height.
- Move your left foot about 30 cm (12 ins) in front of the right foot (Fig.42).

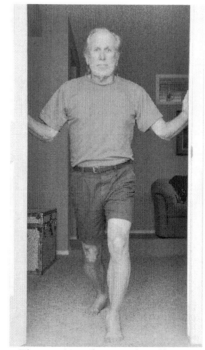

Figure 42. The Heel Pull (a)

- Keep both heels flat on the floor.
- Bend both knees until you feel a pull above the right heel.
- Hold the position for ten seconds.
- You can also rotate your neck while in this position.
- Now switch positions so your right foot is the forward one.
- Bend the knees until you feel the pull above your left heel (Fig. 43).

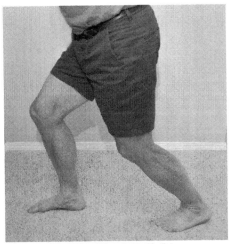

Figure 43. The Heel Pull (b)

- Hold for ten seconds.
- Repeat the stretch five times with each foot.

A variation of this stretch is to keep the back leg straight while you shift your weight to the front leg and bend the front knee. Here you will feel the pull mostly in the back of your calf muscle. The towel stretch is another option that may help if you regularly experience foot pain. Try it just before you get out of bed in the morning. It is easy to do. Sit up in bed with your legs outstretched and a towel wrapped around the ball of one foot. Pull back on the towel hard enough to feel it in your calf muscle and hold for ten seconds. Repeat five or six times with each foot. This will help to loosen up your feet before you get going for the day.

The Shrug

While standing at the doorway, take a moment to work on your shoulders and neck muscles.

- Stand in the middle of the doorway with your feet together.
- Place your hands shoulder high on either side of the outside door frame.
- Lean forward until your arms are straight and your chest is pushed out (Fig.44). The knees and back remain straight (Fig. 45).

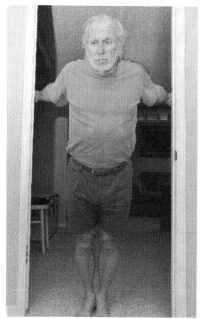 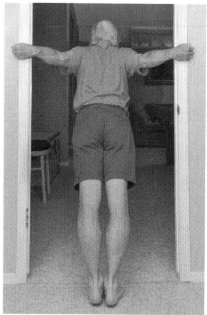

Figure 44. The Shrug (a)   Figure 45. The Shrug (b)

- The pressure should be felt on your shoulders and shoulder blades
- Remain in this position while you rotate your head from side to side.
- Pull halfway back and pause to feel the pressure in your shoulders.
- Hold this position for five seconds.
- Move forward and backward four or five times.

The Yoga Man

The next exercise is good for both your back and your stomach. It also requires good balance, so you may find it a little difficult if this is your first attempt at doing it.

- Get down on the mat on your hands and knees.
- Your thighs should be perpendicular to your calves.
- Extend your right arm shoulder high straight out in front of you.
- Raise your left leg until it is parallel to the floor.
- Squeeze in your stomach muscles.
- Hold the position for seven seconds (Fig. 46).

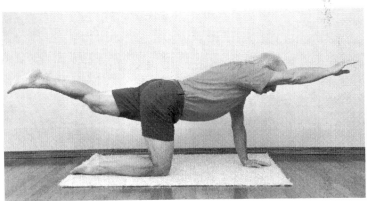

Figure 46. The Yoga Man

- Switch arms and legs and again hold the position for seven seconds.
- Repeat the sequence.
- Now repeat the sequence holding each position for thirty seconds.
- Repeat the sequence again holding each position for seven seconds.

The Back Cruncher & Superman

Be careful. These two stretches can be a strain on the lower back so proceed with caution.

- Lie out on the mat on your stomach.
- Place your hands flat on the mat and push your torso up.
- Keep your legs flat on the floor.
- Straighten the elbows and push down into the mat with your hips.
- Hold the position for ten seconds (Fig. 47).

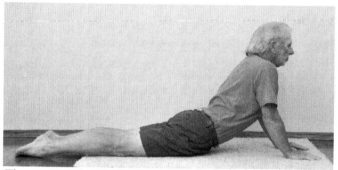

Figure 47. The Back Cruncher

- Now stretch your arms straight out along your head.
- Raise your legs as high as you can while keeping them straight.
- Hold the position for ten seconds (Fig. 48).

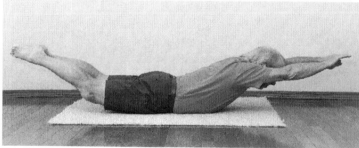

Figure 48. Superman

- Repeat the complete sequence three times.

The Turtle

Our final back stretch is good for loosening the lower back muscles before a game of golf. It also feels good.

- Kneel down on your hands and knees.
- Lean back until your buttocks are resting on your heels.
- Then lean forward with your hands on the floor.
- Keep your butt as close as possible to your heels.
- Reach out as far as you can along the floor with your hands (Fig. 49).

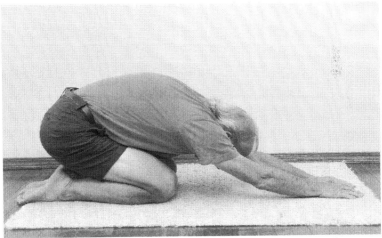

Figure 49. The Turtle

- Hold this position for ten seconds.
- Repeat three times.

Knee Bender

Your workout ends with a challenging exercise to strengthen the knees. The knee consists of the patella (i.e. kneecap) and the joint where the femur and tibia bones are connected by ligaments. The knee joint is the largest joint in our bodies. Our knees have a lot of stress placed on them as we go about our daily activities. This repetitive movement leaves the muscular strength, flexibility and endurance found in healthy knees susceptible to deterioration. However, wear and tear on the knees can be minimized by proper stretching and exercise. You have already worked the knees to some extent with The Leg Twister (Fig. 11), The Toe Grabber (Fig. 17) and the Long John Silver (Fig. 22) stretches, but we take it up a notch with the Knee Bender. Do have a go.

- Kneel down on the mat with your buttocks resting on your heels.
- Place your hands behind you, palms down on the mat.
- Gradually lower your head and torso back toward the mat.
- Keep your knees down on the mat (Fig. 50).

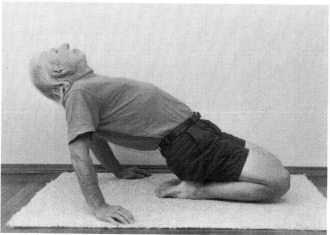

Figure 50. The Knee Bender

48

- Lean back as far as you can without losing your balance or snapping your kneecaps.
- Hold this position for twenty seconds.
- Repeat three times.

This completes the exercise and stretching parts of the program. If you plan to follow this workout routine, I suggest you set up a schedule and stick to it. Everyone has to find his or her own comfort zone in terms of when and how often to work out. There are plenty of options. Some seniors work out in the morning, some later in the day and still others at night. Some go at it six days a week, some like alternate days, while others prefer two days on followed by two days off. The scheduling is up to you. Just be realistic with your planning because a schedule that truly works for you will increase the likelihood of your sticking with the program. I work out five times a week during the winter. I cut it back to three times a week during the golf season but also do an abbreviated routine on the days I am playing golf. I usually work out in the morning. This arrangement works for me but may not for you. It really does not matter. Whatever schedule you can stick to is the one for you.

You also need to decide on the length of your workout. The program outlined here takes about an hour to complete, but the timeline is not set in stone. You can still reap the benefits with a shorter routine. However, there are limits. For example, a fifteen-minute session twice a week will not cut it. For me the minimum is thirty minutes, three times a week, and that is cutting it thin. You also have plenty of choices when it comes to which stretches and exercises to include in a customized program. There is nothing sacred about my selections. However, there are a few guidelines you should observe if you decide to set up your own program. First, do the research needed to ensure your preferred stretches actually do what you think they are doing. Second, it is essential to include both stretching and strengthening exercises in your repertoire. Third, opt for diversity to ensure all parts of your body are put in motion. Finally, leave room for some aerobic conditioning.

Once you reach expert status in this program, you can move onto the Flexi program where you learn to act really silly. This you definitely try at your own risk.

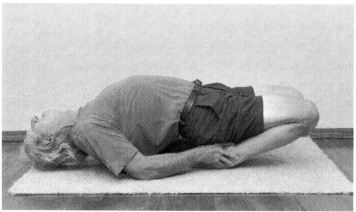
Figure 51. The Flexi Man

Muscle tone, strength and flexibility are key factors when it comes to maintaining an active lifestyle, but you also need a healthy and efficient cardio system if you want to maximize your physical potential. On that note, let us turn our attention to aerobics.

Huffing and Puffing

A erobic exercise or conditioning is an essential component for any top-notch fitness program. The distinguishing characteristic of aerobic exercise is the extra load it puts on your heart and lungs by sustained, rhythmic activity. Aerobic simply means 'with oxygen'. Aerobic exercise calls for your body to use oxygen to help produce the extra energy required during the exercise. This means your heart and lungs are working harder to deliver the oxygen needed throughout your body to continue the exercise. This extra work strengthens the heart and lungs.

There is no debate about the value of aerobic exercise. It is good for you. Indeed it would take a very thick book to report all the scientific evidence showing this to be the case. Here are just a few of the benefits discovered through scientific studies. Aerobic exercise is known to reduce the risk of numerous health problems including high blood pressure, type 2 diabetes, cardiovascular disease and certain kinds of cancer. It also has been shown to have a positive impact on cholesterol levels by lowering low-density lipoprotein (LDL) or 'bad' cholesterol and increasing high-density lipoprotein (HDL) or 'good' cholesterol. It leaves you less susceptible to colds and flu because it activates your immune system, which is used to fight off viral illnesses.[9] It also can help to ward off osteoporosis when the exercise of choice is a weight-bearing one such as walking or running. I am confident you also will feel good and improve your energy levels when you work aerobic exercise into your conditioning program.

The key to aerobic exercise is to be in perpetual motion. The level of intensity and length of time can vary given your personal objectives. My tendency is to be moderate when it comes to intensity and somewhat ambitious with respect to duration. This means my focus is more on

---

[9] It has been at least twenty years since I have had any viral illness. I chalk that up to getting an annual flu shot and regular aerobic exercise.

trying to stick with the activity for a longer period of time rather than worrying about the level of strain usually associated with going faster. So if you are a jogger following this approach, rather than worrying about how fast you are going, you are more concerned with how long you stick at it.

There are a number of activities to choose from when looking for an aerobic workout. Some of the more popular ones are running, biking, cross-country skiing, swimming, snowshoeing, and skating. You also have the option of using stationary equipment such as a treadmill, bicycle or rowing machine. These activities require different skills and the use of different muscle groups, but the common denominator is the workout they give your heart and lungs. Aerobic exercise requires no organization or help from other people. You simply select an activity, get the required equipment and go for it. This works for many people. However, some folks do not have a hope in hell of sticking with an aerobic routine if they try to do it on their own. They need a few friends or some kind of fitness group to keep them going. Well, this is no barrier. If you are an exercising socialite, simply join a group or get two or three friends to work out with you.

Let's look at some of the advantages and disadvantages related to different aerobic activities. This information may prove helpful to those who are trying to decide on an aerobic activity.

Walking. This is the most accessible activity of all. Too often walking is ignored when it comes to aerobic activity, yet it has many advantages. It is a viable option no matter where you hang your hat. Just go outside. It requires no equipment. You can do it alone, with a companion, or as a member of a walking group. Obviously it is a great choice if you have a dog. However, I have one cautionary note. Walking is not a great aerobic exercise if you just saunter along. You have to pick up the pace. An hour walk is a good workout when done at a reasonable pace.

Ice Skating. This is a great way to do your aerobics if you have access to ice. One barrier may be the cost of skates. As well as giving your heart and lungs a workout, it is great exercise for your legs and keeps you working on balance. This is not an activity I would recommend for novices, although if you were a good skater in the past, getting back into it after a long layoff is feasible. Similar to walking, you must remember to keep a good pace and not be taking breaks. For the more ambitious, you cannot beat a game of shinny. A forty-minute skate is a reasonable session.

Jogging. This is probably the most popular aerobic exercise. I was a faithful jogger for about thirty years. I even completed a ten-mile run in seventy-five minutes when I was in my early forties. So I was a keener. However, as I moved into my mid-forties, the lustre wore off. Similar to walking, jogging can be done just about anywhere and requires no special equipment. The downside is the impact it has on your joints. This becomes more of a threat as you age, especially with regard to your knees. Many older men and women have told me they had to stop because of knee or foot pain or both. If you do jog, I urge you to run on soft surfaces in very good runners. A good run can be done in forty minutes.

Cross-Country Skiing. An excellent choice for those who live in a winter climate. The equipment can get expensive, but unlike downhill skiing, you have no lift charges. Most people can find some public land where they can ski for no charge. This is an exercise where you can really challenge your cardiovascular system. It also gives your legs and arms a good workout. A cheaper alternative when it comes to equipment is snowshoeing. Either activity will give your cardiovascular system a good workout if you keep going non-stop for forty-five minutes. Of course, these are not suitable choices if you do not like being outdoors in the winter.

Swimming. Another excellent choice, but it does have a few barriers. For starters, you have to know how to swim reasonably well so you can do thirty or forty laps. Mind you, people do learn to swim later in life, so it is still an option if you are prepared to learn. Access to a pool can also be a barrier for some people because most pools have an admittance charge. The other disadvantage to swimming is crowding. In some pools, finding an open lane can be a challenge. However, these disadvantages aside, there is nothing that beats swimming as an aerobic conditioning exercise. It gives the heart and lungs a great workout and also is fabulous exercise for your arms, legs and feet. The added bonus is the lack of strain on your joints. If it is practically feasible, I would recommend this exercise as the number one choice.

Biking. This has two limitations. The weather has to be reasonably decent, and a bike costs money. However, the bike does not have to be one of the modern mountain bikes costing a couple of grand. The old bike in the garage will serve the purpose so long as it is in running order. The weather is more limiting. You will have to have a second option because cycling is seasonal unless you live in a very moderate climate. Nevertheless, if you have the bike and the weather cooperates, it can be an ideal activity. You get the cardio workout along with leg and knee strengthening. The bottom pedal should be adjusted so that your knee is bent 15/20° to maximize the benefits to your knees. A forty-minute ride at a good pace on a regular road gets the job done.

Using Equipment. Many seniors like to get their exercise on workout machines. This is an option for aerobics. All you need is the machine. Some who can afford it buy a treadmill, stationary bike or rowing machine and work out somewhere in the house. Others get to use machines by joining a health club or a community centre. If you can afford it, like to work out indoors, and are comfortable working up a sweat on a machine, then this is certainly a viable choice. You are good to go with forty minutes of work on any of these machines.

There are other options out there, but I leave it to you to discover them. The important thing is to set up a program that makes working out fun. Enjoying your workout significantly increases the likelihood you will stick at it over the long term. It does not matter if you never exercised in the past or have not done so for years. It is never too late to get started. If you are new to the game, buy into the notion that slow and steady wins the race. Stay in motion.

Want to contact the author? Send an email:
drlarrymcconnell@gmail.com

Read Dr. McConnell's award-winning book on heart disease.
Cardiac Champs
How To Live A Healthy, Vigorous, Happy Life After A Heart Attack
Second Edition 2014

Cardiac Champs is a must read for anyone interested in adopting a realistic plan to control the 'emotional luggage' so often associated with the various forms of heart disease.

Dr. McConnell wisely uses humour and optimism to avoid any cathartic outpouring as he maps out his program to conquer anger, anxiety, panic attacks, insomnia, lifestyle disruptions and the perpetual fear of death. His unique perspective comes through loud and clear when he discusses his approach to physicians, "They are consultants, not managers"; to alcohol, "Enjoy your beer"; and to anger, "Don't get angry, don't get mad, and don't get even."

Readers' comments posted on amazon.com ....

"This book breathes vitality, humor and optimism."

"Doctors should recommend it to their patients".

"Helpful mix of wisdom and humour."   *"An inspirational read."*

"It will provide you with a motivational kick-start..."

"The book provides practical and common sense solutions"

Dr. McConnell's doctoral degree in counselling psychology from McGill University and his thirty-year history with heart disease give him a unique perspective into the psychological effects of living with heart disease, a perspective he says is noticeably absent in treating the disease.

Visit amazon.com (i.e.books) to read more about **Cardiac Champs.**

A Unique Book For Older Men

Dr. Larry McConnell's latest book on living the good life is a must read for every man striving to realize the full potential of his senior years.

A Primer For Old Guys
Eat Smart, Exercise, Be Happy
First Edition 2014

Dr. McConnell embraces the ageing process with good humour and a contagious sense of optimism which is clearly apparent as he expertly motivates his readers to take charge of their physical, psychological and social well-being. No gimmicks. No quick fixes. Just well-researched, practical strategies for maintaining a healthy lifestyle.

Most books directed at seniors tend to focus on exercises or medical issues. This book expands the boundaries as it explores a vast array of issues related to ageing including attitude, nutrition, intimacy, fashion, socializing, finances and grandparenting.

Readers' comments posted on amazon.......

"It is filled with great tips......especially concerning diet and exercise"

"About time somebody with his credentials wrote an easy to read book on this subject for us old dudes."

"Offers common sense and a sense of humor in a practical guide to healthy aging."

"A really positive, but realistic outlook on ageing well."

Written by an old guy for old guys, *A Primer For Old Guys* offers up a comprehensive lifestyle guide that hits all the right buttons with its far-reaching action plan that includes age-appropriate stretching and exercise routines, easy-to-prepare meal recipes, practical budget designs, self-advocacy strategies for dealing with physicians, guidelines for assessing medications as well as professional insights on managing relationships with spouses, children and grandchildren.

Visit amazon.com (books) to read more about **A Primer For Old Guys.**

31810154R00042

Made in the USA
Middletown, DE
12 May 2016